Coping With Cancer

A Patient Pocket Book of Thoughts, Advice, and Inspiration for the Ill

By Veronica Blaha Decker, RN, CNP, MBA,
and Linda Weller-Ferris, BA, MA, PhD

Hygeia Media
An imprint of the Oncology Nursing Society
Pittsburgh, Pennsylvania

ONS Publishing Division
Publisher: Leonard Mafrica, MBA, CAE
Director, Commercial Publishing: Barbara Sigler, RN, MNEd
Managing Editor: Lisa M. George, BA
Technical Content Editor: Angela D. Klimaszewski, RN, MSN
Staff Editor: Amy Nicoletti, BA
Copy Editor: Laura Pinchot, BA
Graphic Designer: Dany Sjoen

Coping With Cancer: A Patient Pocket Book of Thoughts, Advice, and Inspiration for the Ill

First printing, March 2009
Second printing, December 2010

Library of Congress Control Number: 2009923526

ISBN: 978-1-890504-79-3

Publisher's Note
This book is published by the Oncology Nursing Society (ONS). ONS neither represents nor guarantees that the practices described herein will, if followed, ensure safe and effective patient care. The recommendations contained in this book reflect ONS's judgment regarding the state of general knowledge and practice in the field as of the date of publication. The recommendations may not be appropriate for use in all circumstances. Those who use this book should make their own determinations regarding specific safe and appropriate patient-care practices, taking into account the personnel, equipment, and practices available at the hospital or other facility at which they are located. The editors and publisher cannot be held responsible for any liability incurred as a consequence from the use or application of any of the contents of this book. Figures and tables are used as examples only. They are not meant to be all-inclusive, nor do they represent endorsement of any particular institution by ONS. Mention of specific products and opinions related to those products do not indicate or imply endorsement by ONS. Web sites mentioned are provided for information only; the hosts are responsible for their own content and availability. Unless otherwise indicated, dollar amounts reflect U.S. dollars.

ONS publications are originally published in English. Publishers wishing to translate ONS publications must contact the ONS Publishing Division about licensing arrangements. ONS publications cannot be translated without obtaining written permission from ONS. (Individual tables and figures that are reprinted or adapted require additional permission from the original source.) Because translations from English may not always be accurate or precise, ONS disclaims any responsibility for inaccuracies in words or meaning that may occur as a result of the translation. Readers relying on precise information should check the original English version.

Printed in the United States of America

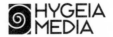

An imprint of the Oncology Nursing Society

With love to my family,
David, Brian, Paul, Marc, and Anne,
for your continuing support, love,
and encouragement.
—*Veronica*

Thanks, Joseph, Robert, and Lindsey,
for your endless patience with my work,
words of encouragement, creative insights,
and little pushes to get this project out.
I love you!
—*Linda*

Contents

Introduction

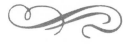

You often hear people say that health is the greatest human blessing. When you are diagnosed with a serious or chronic illness, you understand how easy it is to take your health for granted. When a doctor gives you news of a serious diagnosis, you find yourself suddenly trapped in a crisis situation—one that challenges even the strongest and bravest. Illness changes your entire life in an instant. From that moment on, your thoughts, routines, self-concept, and goals change. Your work life changes. Family life changes. You grapple with managing the immediate crisis—the diagnosis of your illness and decisions about its treatment. Then you move on to managing doctors, family members, friends, bosses, and coworkers.

This book will give you knowledge, insight, and good judgment in many of the situations you now face. When you are in tough circumstances, you can look to this book to find just the right words. As you face treatments and physical struggles, this book will help you to manage your private thoughts and emotions. This book will give you some operating principles that will guide you through challenging physical times. It will show you how to replace negatives with positives, like conflict with harmony, crisis with stability, inactivity with activity, depression with hope, and secrecy with openness.

That's what this book is: coping strategies for anyone who is ill. It is a pocket book that will advise you on a variety of social and psychological issues as you combat illness. In the worst of times, you'll be able to find simple words of advice to get you through. When you're feeling overwhelmed, this book will give you a more positive perspective. The diagnosis of an illness puts you into new territory, and sometimes it is difficult to get your bearings. Many times, you're stumped over how to work through a problem.

This tiny book is packed with invaluable insight and numerous ways to cope with serious and chronic illness. It lends perspective, good judgment, and advice—sometimes with a touch of humor—to anyone who is ill. It gives you hints on finding one-minute pleasures, sustaining hope, and creating positive thoughts. It is packed with tips on coping. This book is your gift from the thousands of ill patients we have counseled over the decades. You can witness the miracle of a quality life despite illness.

With love,

Veronica Blaha Decker, RN, CNP, MBA
Linda Weller-Ferris, BA, MA, PhD

1

Diagnosis

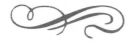

Knowledge	All patients have their most stressful time within the first six months of diagnosis.
Tell Yourself	"I can and will improve my life from here on out. I'll use this experience as my wake-up call."

You have the right to feel shock, disappointment, fear, self-pity, and anxiety. Consider doing the following.

→ Try using the "worry clock" exercise. Set a timer, such as a handheld cooking timer or an oven timer. Any amount of time on the clock is fine, although we suggest limiting the time to 10–15 minutes when you first start using this exercise. Pull out a sheet of paper and make a list of your worries, from most to least worrisome. In a second column, identify whether this worry is under your control, uncontrollable, or if you may take some action to partially control or affect the issue worrying you. If a worry is uncontrollable, and you cannot do anything to affect the source of the problem or the outcome, then strike it from the list. You should direct your attention and energy toward those issues that you may influence or control. In the last column, list all the actions that you could take to alleviate or lessen a worry. This exercise gives you direction and purpose. People who use it find that it lessens their depression and feelings of helplessness. Once the timer rings, you must leave the worry list until the following day. If you find your thoughts drifting to a concern during the day, tell yourself that you are off the worry clock and that you can devote time and energy to that concern tomorrow. Each day, you can evaluate your list and action items, adding to it and deleting from it. So, when the timer goes off, you're done! Dry your tears. Compose yourself. Seal off your worries, and get up and go on to a productive activity—one that pleases you and gives you self-satisfaction and a feeling of accomplishment.

→ Throughout the day, if you find yourself slipping back into negative thoughts, worries, or emotions, tell yourself that you've spent enough time and energy worrying and sorting through those issues today. You can go back on the worry clock tomorrow.

→ Crying and feeling sorry for oneself is a common initial reaction to serious health issues. Remember to do this for no more than 10–20 minutes per day. Although it is important to acknowledge and allow yourself to have those emotions, maintaining your normal life routine as much as you are physically able to is more important.

→ Most people find it helpful to begin a journal. Purchase a small notebook, and write out your story about this health problem. Start the journal at the point when you began feeling ill and experiencing symptoms. Write all the details surrounding your diagnosis. Write about your emotions, fears, anxieties, and stresses. This journal helps you to work through your emotions and worries. Keep this as a private diary of your struggles and issues with illness.

→ No one ever says, "Gee, I wish I would have worried more." Worrying or thinking the worst does not help you to get through this crisis, nor does it bring you joy. The goal is to be productive and happy, despite this illness.

→ Remember: Allow yourself a maximum of 30 minutes a day to feel sad and down about this illness. Then, get on with living.

2

Crisis Management

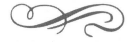

Knowledge	The diagnosis of an illness is a personal crisis.
Tell Yourself	"I am handling my diagnosis like a crisis situation! Discretion is of the highest order."

Think about the following.

✦ Remember that you have both the right and the responsibility to manage information about your illness and its treatment. It's your problem, and you should manage it.

✦ You must decide who you wish to tell about your diagnosis. Remember that this is *your* choice. You do not have to disclose it to everyone. You may be selective.

✦ Think about the ramifications of this knowledge regarding your health situation.

✦ Tell those who will give you support, guidance, help, and knowledge. Tell those who are intimately a part of your life. Secrecy builds walls and barriers between people. Tell those you live with about your diagnosis. Use simple and direct language that they will understand. Be open about any changes that may be occurring in your relationship with them as you go through treatment for your illness. This is never comfortable, but openness takes away anxieties and fears that result from secrecy.

✦ Always tell your immediate family and closest friends about your diagnosis. Be totally open with the people who are most significant in your life. Secrets prevent closeness.

✦ What do you tell others about the diagnosis? Remember that you do not have to disclose the details of your diagnosis and treatment to everyone.

✦ Tell your boss only as much as needed to explain medical absences or leaves. Most bosses are compassionate and understanding, but some are not. Telling people at work about your illness can be a sensitive matter, and unfortunately, public knowledge of a person's illness has been known to damage careers. Ask yourself if you *really* want coworkers to know personal information, for example, if you have breast, gynecologic, or prostate problems. Think this through. Consider the ramifications of sharing this information with people beforehand, not after. You can easily offer vague yet seemingly open disclosures when talking about an illness with coworkers.

→ You can choose to be discreet.

→ You can use ignorance as a defense to others' questions. Saying you don't know or changing the subject can get you out of uncomfortable conversations.

→ Remember, too, that you can choose *when* you tell others about a diagnosis. So, as the saying goes, "timing is everything." A key to successful illness management is being prepared to deal with others successfully. You don't need added stress, worry, and anxiety. Preparation is important, so take the time for it.

→ Also remember that you are the priority right now. When you find yourself too focused on taking care of everybody else's feelings and reactions to your illness, it may be time to step back and take a break. You need to devote a majority of your energy to stabilizing your health and daily routine, not caring for the emotional and psychological needs of others. You should periodically monitor how much catering and concern you are giving to others surrounding *their* handling of *your* diagnosis. After all, you are the one who is ill. Step back.

Give others the time and space needed to react on their own to your diagnosis. Let them work it out for themselves for a while.

✦ Continually ask yourself what *you* want. With whom do you want to share intimate details of your journey? Be certain that the choices are yours.

✦ Boundaries are healthy. Define yours clearly. You are the one struggling to get better. If others intrude on your privacy, tell them politely that you would prefer not to discuss certain issues.

✦ Learn to give nondescript yet socially acceptable answers to questions about your health, such as
  - "I'm doing fine."
  - "I'm feeling good enough to be here!"
  - "I'm feeling fine. I take one day at a time now."
  - "I'm a fighter."
  - "I live in the here and now."

✦ Some patients have used shockers, such as "I'm not dead yet, so relax!" This is another style issue for you to sort through.

3

Doctor's Visits

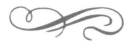

Knowledge	Most patients are overwhelmed by their diagnosis and are afraid of the disease. Some may feel intimidated by doctors. As a result, many patients forget to ask them important questions.
Tell Yourself	"I can get the information I want from this doctor. After all, we all put our clothes on the same way, and I'm paying the bill!"

You are not alone if doctors intimidate you. However, they are powerful people in your fight to get better, and the success of your relationship is important and necessary. Remember the following.

✦ Write down all your questions before every visit to the doctor. It may take you a day or two to remember everything you want to ask. Keep an ongoing list.

→ Ask the following kinds of questions.

- Tell me all about this illness. Would you please describe it to me in simple, biologic terms?
- What caused it?
- What are the symptoms of this illness?
- How might it progress?
- How is it treated? (When, where, and why does the treatment work?)
- What are the side effects of the treatment?
- Can my illness be cured or stopped?
- What if I don't respond to the first treatment efforts? Do other treatments exist for this illness?
- What's the prognosis of this illness? (This is an optional question that you should ask only if you want to know.)

→ No question is a stupid question. If a question pops into your mind, ask it.

→ Tell yourself to listen to the doctor. Focus on thinking about what the doctor is saying in response to your questions. You do not have to worry about formulating the next question, because you have written them down ahead of time.

→ Repeat or paraphrase what the doctor is saying to make sure that you understand the information.

→ If you do not understand what the doctor is saying, then ask him or her to explain the terms. Feel free to ask the doctor to review it one more time.

→ Take notes. Write down the answers to your questions. You may opt to record the session on audiotape. Most oncologists understand a request to tape record a meeting with them in which they are providing new and often complex information; however, it's always a good idea to ask before recording.

→ Ask for written information about your illness. Don't let communication problems prevent you from learning about your illness and its treatments. If your doctor is foreign-born and you cannot decipher his English, then ask for a nurse to help.

→ Ask the doctor to recommend books or references about your illness. However, it is okay if you don't want information about your illness. We have found that approximately 70% of patients feel in greater control and cope better if they have some basic information about their illness, but about 30% find that information about their illness creates higher levels of anxiety and depression. The need for information is not related to the educational level of a person, either.

→ Most patients have the problem of *listening to but not hearing* what their doctor is saying. For example, one patient admitted that once the doctor gave her the diagnosis, she sat there nodding her head in agreement, as though she agreed with what the doctor was saying. In reality, she was thinking, "Gee, I'd like to fix her hair." Take a friend or family member with you to your initial appointments. They can be good listeners and can help to recall details and interpret information for you after the visit is over. Be careful that you choose the most appropriate person for the job. Don't choose nosy, opinionated, negative, or overly emotional people for this job.

✦ It usually is prudent and advisable to seek a second opinion about your diagnosis and treatment. Some patients look for several treatment options. This will depend upon your treatment decision-making style and preference.

4

Treatment Decisions

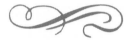

Knowledge	Treatment decisions require knowledge, self-assurance, courage, and inquisitiveness. Treatment decision making is an important part of managing most illnesses.
Tell Yourself	"I have the confidence, courage, time, and talent to make good decisions. I will gain knowledge about my treatment options so that I will make sound treatment decisions."

Treatment decisions are part of any battle against illness. More and more often, treatment decisions are placed with patients. Patients take many different approaches to making decisions about treatment. Some patients never seek a second opinion. They take the diagnosis and treatment recommendation from one doctor and leave it at that. Others immediately seek multiple medical opinions, even just to confirm the diagnosis. Here are a few tips to get you through this.

→ In almost all cases, you should seek a second opinion. Wide variations may exist in the treatment of your illness.

→ Don't get anxious because of a *false sense of urgency*. In most cases, you have time to locate another reputable doctor and set up an appointment. Seek the information you deserve.

→ Make your own health chart to summarize all the information from different doctors. Write down the diagnosis, treatment, drugs, drug dosages, and frequency and duration of treatment. The key is to find a comfortable way to look at all the information from different doctors so that you can easily compare them. Ask about side effects and possible complications. Don't expect to get 12 years of medical training in two weeks. You don't have to be the medical expert; you just have to know how to choose expert medical care.

→ Ask doctors "why" questions. Ask questions such as "Why are you suggesting that we treat my illness this way?" and "What is the standard of care for my illness?"

→ Once you have agreement from at least two doctors on your diagnosis and treatment, it is important to comply with those recommendations. Although treatments may be challenging, painful, or disruptive to your life, you should understand that the treatments are probably necessary for a cure and your survival. If you are having trouble forming the courage to have a treatment, refer to Chapter 2 and Chapter 9 of this book. As therapists, we usually are successful in getting patients through the treatments.

→ What happens when doctors have different approaches to the treatment of your illness? You should weigh their data, training, reputation, and documented outcomes of treatments. Asking doctors why they are making treatment recommendations is the key here. Have the courage to probe a doctor when you see obvious differences of opinion. Remember that it is your body and your life.

→ Make sure that your treatment decisions are not based on faulty medical beliefs about how your body systems really work. Ask questions of your doctor in order to check that your prior knowledge is medically accurate.

→ Some experimental treatments are terribly expensive and not covered by medical insurance companies. You need to carefully weigh the medical data—not your emotions. You could be bankrupting your family needlessly. Don't slip into the easy trap of saying, "If you love me, you'll pay for this treatment!"

➔ When you and your family disagree over your treatment decisions, you should take the time to figure out why. Do they have valid concerns? Have you evaluated the medical information in the same way? Do you and your family members have the same goals and values surrounding your treatment? Keep your communications open. You most likely will need their support to get through the physical realities of some treatments, such as transportation and physical companionship.

➔ Remember that many family conflicts surrounding treatment decisions occur over a patient's choice to continue or discontinue treatments. It is ultimately your choice; however, be careful to listen to family members' worries, opinions, and concerns.

➔ It may be important to reaffirm treatment decisions periodically by continuing to learn about your disease and its treatment.

➔ Don't let friends or families undermine your decisions.

➔ Remember that you didn't ask for this illness. Treatments should not be viewed as your deserved suffering.

➔ Painful, debilitating treatments are not a path of forgiveness from God. Seek spiritual guidance if you find yourself thinking this way.

✦ Don't relinquish your sense of power and responsibility for your treatment decisions. They should be yours, and not that of others. The more you participate in your treatment decisions, the more ownership you will feel. You will also hold greater confidence in how things will turn out. Seize this as an opportunity to take control of your illness. Answer your illness with sound treatments!

5

Understanding Common Issues

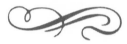

Knowledge	Comparing your reactions, problems, and challenges with others suffering from the same illness is initially reassuring. It can help you feel that you are not alone, and your reactions and worries are not outside the norm.
Tell Yourself	"It is normal to compare myself to others who have this illness. My reactions, issues, and problems are common to everyone struggling with this illness. I'm not going crazy. I can and will find ways to gain control of my life, reactions, and emotions. I must be careful not to get stuck in a rut of endless comparison and must focus on taking charge of my life in relation to this illness."

Comparing our lives to others' is an everyday event for us. Whenever we go through new experiences, we tend to measure our experience against other people's. The reactions and issues associated with any serious or chronic illness typically follow patterns. Prior knowledge about those patterns allows you to more easily calm yourself and feel at ease.

The following list summarizes the most common things you'll have to conquer.

→ A fear of death itself because of the uncertainty of what lies beyond

→ A fear of the dying processes. Although you may have a deep faith in God or a higher power, you fear the pain, suffering, physical deterioration, and physical dependency associated with death.

→ Not wanting to leave your life on earth. You feel cheated out of life's time and events with those you love.

→ Physical problems associated with your condition or the medical treatments for your condition

→ Losing or gaining weight. Remember: If you couldn't eat Twinkies® and hot fudge sundaes without gaining weight before you became ill, you probably can't now! Also remember that weight loss is an equally difficult battle for others, too.

→ Feeling so anxious and upset that you cannot concentrate on anything for a long period of time

✦ Forgetfulness that intrudes on your quality of life

✦ Depression that includes symptoms such as loss of appetite, sleep problems, sadness, crying, an inability to get things done, or a lethargic reaction to your activities

✦ A constant preoccupation with your body functions and how you are feeling physically; worrying that the illness is worsening or spreading

✦ Problems managing work demands because of worry or physical limitations

✦ Problems meeting demands in your home life, such as cooking, cleaning, shopping, or laundry

✦ Problems with your social relationships. You may limit your social contacts or change living arrangements because of illness.

✦ Problems with your sexuality. Expect to be less interested in sex when you are worried about dying! You also may have body image issues as a result of treatments or surgeries.

✦ You may be preoccupied with time. How much longer to live? How long will I feel this way? How much longer will treatments go on? It can become an obsession. A woman with leukemia had a new roof put on her house, and the roofer proudly announced that her roof should last her another 20 years. The woman burst into tears, saying, "Great, but will I?"

✦ Chemotherapy patients have a very difficult time with hair loss. It is a painful reminder of one's condition, and a public one at that.

✦ You may have intense anxiety or dread over your medical treatments. Treatments such as dialysis, cardiac rehabilitation, chemotherapy, and even chronic insulin injections may cause you emotional turmoil and worry. You are not alone if you have these reactions.

6

Defining Your Adversities

Knowledge	Most adults have complicated, fast-paced, demanding lives. When illness strikes, you will face some adversities. You'll have to make adjustments in your lifestyle. Common personal issues and social dilemmas arise. Define your adversities right from the point of diagnosis.
Tell Yourself	"I will sort through and understand the meaning of this illness in terms of my life—family, work, friends, and finances. I can successfully manage and respond to the ramifications of this illness. I'm adaptive!"

You need to step back and take a fresh look at your life. Allow yourself the time and psychological space necessary to define the adversities that you face. You have a unique life—one that is made up of home, work, and relationships. The problems this illness causes you most often are not the only concerns you have going on in your life. The kind of adversity and how much challenge you face depends on your life-style *right now*. Perform the following steps in order to put this illness within the context of your life. Ask yourself the following questions, and write your responses in your journal.

→ "What does this illness mean to my relationship with my most significant companions? How will they cope with this illness? How will they react? In what ways will this illness impact our relationships and lifestyle?"

→ If you have children, ask yourself these questions: "What does this illness mean to my children? How will this illness affect them? Have I given them enough or too much information about my illness?"

→ "What does this illness do to my work life?"

→ "What does this illness mean to my friends?"

→ "Am I expressing confidence to others that my treatment decisions are sound?"

→ "Have I recognized the challenges associated with my illness so that I can make plans to address them?"

A few other issues also are important to remember:

→ Expect to react emotionally. Regardless of a good or bad prognosis, all people have emotional ups and downs at first.

→ There's no "right" way to react to your illness. Despite popular writings, your feelings will *not* follow set "stages." You will find yourself moving in and out of openness and isolation, anger and acceptance, depression and optimism.

→ Know that your initial reactions do not determine, nor predict, how well you will ultimately cope with this illness.

→ Know that the individuals who are most successful at coping with illness make immediate changes in their lifestyles and, over time, come to accept the changes.

→ Know that patients who adjust successfully take actions to manage work demands in order to maintain maximal productivity while giving their bodies the rest they need to heal. You may have to delegate, put off, or cut back on work for a while.

→ Project changes in finances and health insurance, and plan around these issues, too. Ask family members or close friends for short-term financial assistance if you need it. You may have to spend some time developing a viable financial plan for this. Ask for some help in this area.

7

Building a Vision of Your Future

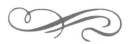

Knowledge	You are the master of your fate. In order to make a road map, you must know where you are going. Illness gives everyone a wake-up call. This experience gives you an opportunity to change aspects of your life for the better. You can now reflectively manage your life. You can make active choices.
Tell Yourself	"I will take control of my life in relation to this illness and its treatments. I will set my course and stay firm. I am the architect of my daily life and my activities. I can transform those aspects of my everyday routines that I find troubling or dissatisfying."

You need to step back and take a fresh look at your life in relation to this illness and its treatments. Although you have already defined your unique challenges, you must know where you want to go in order to figure out how to get there. You should restructure your everyday life to realize your plan.

✦ Daydream: Use your daydreams to get in touch with your creativity. Daydreams have the potential to lend valuable clues as to how you would like things to be. Remember that you want to manage your problems so that they don't manage you.

✦ Use your imagination when thinking about work, home, family, and relationships.

✦ Think about how you might eliminate the negatives in your life.

✦ Focus on how you might build on the positives in your life.

✦ Answer the following questions. You may want to write your answers in your journal.
  - "What do I believe to be my life mission?" (*Life mission* refers to those things that you value most—family, work, volunteer activities, religion, social commitments, etc.)
  - "Why do I value these activities?"
  - "What are my most important daily purposes? Why?"

- "What do I need in order to continue or begin to accomplish my activities?"
- "Can I realistically continue to meet these daily activities?"
- "If I could change one thing about my life before my illness, what would it be? Why?"
- "How might I specifically go about changing it now?"
- "What forces help me to change?"
- "What forces prevent me from changing?"
- "If I could change one thing about my life after my acute illness, what would it be?"

→ Quickly complete the following questions.

- "I am most confused by_____ ."
- "I am most frustrated by_____ ."
- "I am most fearful of_____ ."
- "I feel guilty about _____ ."
- "I feel most angry about_____ ."
- "I feel like a kid again when I _____ ."
- "I get excited when I think about_____ ."
- "I laugh when_____ ."
- "I am curious about _____ ."
- "I am at peace when_____ ."

- "I am happiest when_____ ."

- "I am most fulfilled when_____ ."

- "After I start to feel better, the first thing that I'm going to do is _____ ."

✦ Look over your answers, and decide on the issues that surface. Define one negative thing in your life that you are going to eliminate. Define one positive thing in your life that you are going to enhance.

✦ All your energy and behaviors should be directed toward the positives that you just wrote about.

✦ Follow your dreams and your heart, and you'll become energized and productive, despite illness.

✦ Make yourself a *dream board*. Make a poster and fill it with lists, pictures, maps, and travel brochures that point you toward the future. Dreaming about a future party, get-together, special occasion, or trip to a pleasurable destination is important. When you feel down, just look at your dream board.

8

Proven Ways to Cope

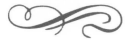

Knowledge	You have the choice to cope well with illness or to cope poorly. You have the answers within.
Tell Yourself	"I will face each day as an opportunity to conquer the effects of illness and its treatments. I will make good coping choices so that I am productive, happy, and at peace."

People use common behaviors to cope with the effects of illness. Some coping choices are better than others; that is, you get more benefit from them. If you want to maintain the most productive and fulfilled life possible, consider doing the following.

✦ Exert personal effort each day, even by the hour. Set goals, and take action to reach your goal. Use your physical and mental energies to do something, great or small. Do things such as reading a book, making a telephone call, writing a letter, reviewing work files, listening to tapes, or ironing some clothes. Your time, strength, and faculties are there to be used.

✦ Exercise. Physical activity increases your physiologic and metabolic responses. Exercising will help you. You do not have to join a health club—just walk around the block. Walk from room to room. Set a daily exercise goal and do it. You'll feel better physically and will likely sleep better, too.

✦ Train in a technique. Learning meditation, relaxation, or imaging techniques will help you feel better as well.

✦ Focus on creating thoughts that you are a person who can cope with adversity.

✦ When depressing thoughts creep into your mind or negative events occur, counter them with a personal resolve to meet the challenge. We know from experience that patients can maintain a decent quality of life with personal effort.

✦ Turn to your family for physical and emotional support. Reliance on family is the most commonly used support mechanism of chronically ill patients. Be careful to pick the best family members for the job.

➤ Friends can pick up your spirits and help you to escape your troubles and preoccupations for a while. Friends can help you physically, too. Pick the most capable ones for physical support. Accept their help, and have the strength to say no to those who cause you stress or worry.

➤ Consider a diet change or healthier eating and drinking choices. This will give you a sense of control over your illness. Quit smoking if you can. These are proven ways to improve your spirits.

➤ Seek information about your illness only if information is a source of comfort for you. Information can be a valuable tool for coping with illness, but not if it generates more worry and depression. Individuals vary greatly regarding how they value and use medical information, and this is not related to one's educational background. You may find that greater information about your illness helps you emotionally and psychologically; however, you may be a person who becomes increasingly distressed and depressed when reading about your illness. You must be the sole judge of the effects of medical information on your overall adjustment.

➤ Don't focus on your prognosis. It is an arbitrary number that may be comforting or distressing to you. Let it go for now.

→ Move to control the consequences of this illness on your lifestyle. Give this serious thought. Ask yourself if you are becoming too isolated and whether you have too many changes in your life. Then make a plan.

→ If you believe that you have somehow caused your illness, then take proactive steps to address this faulty reasoning.

→ Forget support groups for now. You may be lucky enough to find a support group that is a good fit for you; however, be careful not to become depressed, overwhelmed, saddened, and self-pitying as a result of a support group. Many support groups are dumping grounds for woes. Support groups are highly variable in terms of mission, leadership, and participants. Make sure that you know the goals and intent of the group, as well as the credentials of the leader. Our research found that a majority of people join support groups for information about their illness; however, most support groups are not structured to meet this need for information. You may be able to get the information you desire in more effective ways.

→ Don't hug your doctor. Your medical doctor is not your best friend, nor is he or she your psychiatrist. For example, a patient asked an oncologist if he would be the patient's friend. The oncologist was puzzled and said, "If you think I'm going out to have a beer with you, I'm not. If you mean will I be there for you when you get sick, I will." That's what works best—your doctor will be there for you medically when you need him or her.

→ Look for a doctor who gives you the medical information you request, who is hopeful, and who takes the time to communicate with you about your medical issues. Look for a competent physician who is apprised of the state-of-the-art treatment strategies. Look for a doctor whom you like. Look for a doctor who is comfortable with your communication style.

→ Focus on yourself and your needs. Use as many self-directed coping behaviors as possible.

→ You have the answers to your daily happiness. Don't look for rescue from others; you will be sadly disappointed. This is a private battle, and the quality of life achieved is ultimately your responsibility, not that of others around you.

9

Coping With Treatments and Medical Tests

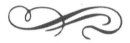

Knowledge   Known ways exist for how to best manage your anxiety, worry, and responses to medical treatments and tests.

Tell Yourself   "I have the tools and personal strength to get through this test or treatment. I can use many of these tips to cope with these medical tests and treatments. I must undergo these procedures for better health. I can do this!"

You are not alone if you are coping with physical problems and emotional reactions as a result of medical tests or treatments. A majority of patients have signifi-

39

cant anxiety, fear, and worry over tests and treatments. You are not alone if you are feeling any of these emotions. A majority of patients also have to cope with negative side effects from treatments. Because we are great learners, our body and psyche naturally want to avoid or escape physically challenging treatments that make us ill. The key is to take steps to minimize your emotional reactions and to manage any side effects from treatments. Consider doing the following.

→ Put your thoughts and worries about upcoming tests and treatments out of your mind. When your thoughts drift there, you must block them and get busy with other activities you enjoy.

→ Tell yourself not to waste energy on this right now. You will deal with it when the test or treatment comes.

→ Tell yourself to take one day at a time.

→ Tell yourself that you *must, can,* and *will* get through the test or the treatment. Continually repeat this to yourself, especially when you find your thoughts drifting into worry.

→ The day before a test or treatment, you should prepare yourself. Do the following.

  – Get your clothes packed, if needed. Do not always wear the same outfit to treatments. You don't want to associate any one outfit with pain, nausea, or fear.

- Select a book to read. Make a selection that will calm you or put you to sleep. Again, don't always read the same book.

- Consider taking a portable music player to your appointment. Pick out a different selection each time. Again, it should be restful and peaceful. Always vary the music. You don't want to hear a song in the future that you associate with a stressful test or punishing treatment. We've seen chemotherapy patients vomit in hallways when they see a nurse or hear certain music they had played over and over. This is called a conditioned response, and you don't want to create one.

- If you've been doing relaxation exercises successfully, you should be prepared to use the recording or apply the principles if you become anxious.

- Plan the foods that you will eat before and after the test or treatment. Again, always vary the foods at these times in order to avoid a conditioned response. Variation is the key to success here.

- Plan your transportation. Ask for a ride. If you tend to get sick in the car, prepare for this, but don't dwell on it or expect it. Tell yourself that you probably won't need these items, but at least you are prepared.

- Always vary your driving route to the hospital or clinic. You don't want to associate landmarks, roads, or routes with pain, panic, or nausea.

– Remember to reward yourself. The day before and the day after a treatment, do something extra-special. Go out to lunch with friends. Eat a favorite snack or treat. Use the operating principle of replacing pain with pleasure.

→ Always have things ready at home for your return from the test or treatment. Have the nightgown out, the house in order, and your bed prepared. Know that you are returning to the comforts of your own home—comforts specific to you.

→ Be careful not to add the demands of your treatments to an already packed agenda. Delegate some commitments or say no so that you can recuperate without worry or added tensions.

→ Plan a reward for getting through this. Tell yourself that if you manage this well, you are going to give yourself a big treat the next day or the following week. Identify something that will be a real reward.

→ Always use the premedications that your doctor prescribes to minimize side effects. There are no rewards for being macho or a silent sufferer. Modern medicine has given us many tools to minimize your discomfort. If you're an "anti-medication" person, tell yourself that you are only using the drugs for a short while. Medications can really help you to get through this. As we tell our patients, "Take the pill!"

10

One-Minute Self-Affirmations

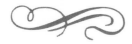

Knowledge	Your thoughts and beliefs direct your behaviors and, therefore, the quality of life you will achieve. How you think about your illness will have a powerful effect on your life.
Tell Yourself	"I can control my thoughts and outlook on this illness. I can affirm myself throughout my day."

You most likely have a secretly held belief about why you got sick. The meaning that you give to your illness is your reality. You should be careful to manage this belief. It will shape your course of action regarding your illness. Your thoughts about your illness and beliefs about its cause also will shape your behaviors. Both your thoughts and behaviors influence how you feel. Feelings such as joy, happiness, pride, sadness, anger, anxiety, and shame may come from either your thoughts or actions. To control your thoughts that create negative feelings, try repeating the following affirmations.

↦ "I can cope."

↦ "I can make compromises in my lifestyle in order to heal."

↦ "I can manage my pain successfully."

↦ "I am a strong person."

↦ "I will conquer negative beliefs about this illness."

↦ "I will overcome this adversity."

↦ "I have faith and trust in my ability to cope."

↦ "I will successfully manage this illness."

↦ "I can get through this medical test."

↦ "I am prepared for whatever comes."

↦ "I will find strength and courage to fight the effects of this illness."

↦ "It is my choice to handle the effects of this illness with dignity and resistance."

↦ "I am able to maintain control and respond appropriately to this illness."

✦ "I am confident with this treatment."

✦ "I can manage my daily life and its demands."

✦ "I must and will exert effort to be productive during my treatments."

✦ "I believe in myself."

✦ "I trust my inner strengths as a person and know that I am capable of managing this illness."

✦ "I can accomplish one meaningful task each day."

✦ "I can depend on others close to me to help me through this rough time."

✦ "I can delegate work, and the world won't end."

✦ "Most housework can wait."

✦ "I can find peacefulness within my own resolve to conquer this illness."

✦ "I am prepared for whatever comes my way."

✦ "I will manage this experience well, for my good and the good of all whom I love."

11

Simple Pleasures

Knowledge	Always replace pain with pleasure.
Tell Yourself	"Life is short. Why suffer, when I can create a happy, pleasurable moment?"

You may have gotten the notion that you need to get in touch with the seriousness of your illness and that you should have to contemplate the meaning of everything now that you are ill. We encourage you to review your priorities (e.g., family, friends, work) in relation to your illness and then make changes where you want. Focusing on your illness and its negative impact on your life is not productive, necessary, or positive. You can get through this illness very well without believing that you need to have intensive psychotherapy or gut-wrenching self-absorption! You can take control of your daily life now and find ways to transcend the negatives associated with illness.

✦ Defiance of the havoc that illness brings is not denial of your illness.

✦ Constantly focusing on your losses because of illness doesn't help you to achieve a better quality of life.

✦ When you find your thoughts drifting to self-pity, get busy. Tell yourself to focus on something else that is positive and productive. If you must, go back to your worry list for a brief time, and then let it go for the day.

✦ You truly create your own quality of life. Unfortunately, no one can do that for you.

✦ Only you can manage your physical pain. Call or consult with your doctor if you are suffering. Effective pain management programs are available for severely ill patients. Don't suffer. Modern pharmaceuticals can alleviate pain and restore your energy and positive attitude.

✦ Consciously tell yourself that you must also manage your emotional pain in some way. Refer to other sections of this book to find a path that works for you.

✦ These are proven simple pleasures for patients:
  - Exercise.
  - Meditate.
  - Telephone a friend or family member.
  - Write in a journal.

- Eat a food you love.
- Snuggle with your pet.
- Accomplish one task you value.
- Write a letter.
- Review a file from work.
- Read a book.
- Listen to music.
- Pray, if you are religious.
- Allow yourself rest if your body craves it.
- Go out to lunch.
- Watch a movie you love.
- Laugh as much as you can.
- Bake or cook something for someone else.
- Learn something new.
- Get on a computer and get lost on the Internet.
- Go to the library.
- Go to a museum or art gallery.
- Garden.
- Read the newspaper or a magazine.
- Go for a walk or run.
- Get busy with your favorite hobby.
- Clean a closet or drawer.
- Watch a favorite TV show.
- Set one goal and do it. Accomplishments feel great!

✦ Avoid such things as

- Negative friends or family members
- The news at bedtime

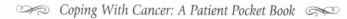

- Dwelling on your problems, illness, limitations, or bodily symptoms
- Lethargy
- Self-pity
- Depressing music
- Tear-jerk movies
- Focusing on your prognosis
- Talk shows that warp your perspective

12

Family

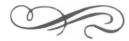

Knowledge	Patients turn to their families in order to cope with chronic or serious illness. Dependence on family is the most widely used coping mechanism by seriously or chronically ill people. You, too, will most likely have to depend on your family for physical, emotional, and social support. Remember that every family has highly functional and dysfunctional parts to it. The key is to manage these relationships.
Tell Yourself	"I can and will find the best ways to get family support during my illness. I must be patient with my family and continually communicate with them about this experience. I must use the insight I have about their styles and personalities to maximize the positive qualities of my family members. I can shape and change relationships with family members."

There is no such thing as a perfect family. Every family has highly functional and dysfunctional parts to it. It is your responsibility to understand both what you need from your family and how you are going to get those things. If you are like most people, you're going to have to manage these relationships, or you will likely find yourself drifting under their control. You also may feel emotionally upset or angry. Your chronic or serious illness will do strange things to other people, especially to family members. Your family members are very likely to experience your reactions of anger, fear, anxiety, sadness, or depression, too. Don't be surprised if you see off-the-wall behaviors. Family members are likely to say stupid things and sometimes behave badly; so, expect it.

The first thing that family members are likely to do is to ask, "*Why?* Why did you get this illness?" Understand that family members may make judgmental statements regarding your diagnosis of illness, and these comments may hurt your feelings. They may directly or indirectly believe that you are somehow responsible for your illness. They may exaggerate the predictability of your diagnosis and say that you should have seen this coming. They may actually degrade you in order to hold on to their sense that it is a just world. You have two choices here: confront or ignore. Many patients successfully confront the person's judgment and protest it. You may feel better doing this; however, you may be sacrificing a relationship, too. Others choose to ignore these comments or beliefs. Some avoid the person. This is a matter of both personal style and how much energy you have to devote to this. Remember that it is your experience. You don't want to act hastily. Cool down. Give it some thought.

You'll want to figure out what you want and need from your family. What kinds of physical support do you require? What kinds of emotional and psychological support do you want? Looking at all the adjustments you must make, where might your family help out? Once you understand *what* you would like from your family regarding support, you must figure out *if* they are actually capable of giving it to you.

Situations may sour in a couple of ways. First, a family may be in a position to help, but doesn't. This is not as rare as it sounds. When families don't pitch in to help you when they could, it will likely cause you hurt feelings and disappointment. Brush it off. You could wallow away in self-pity, anger, and disappointment, but you've got enough problems as it is. Don't create more for yourself. Go back to the drawing board and figure out who may be in a position to help. If family can't, perhaps friends, church members, or coworkers could. The key is not to be surprised if your family is not in a position to help you as much as you'd like. Most patients find that they are surprised as to who helps them and who drops out of the scene.

Second, families burn out. Your family may not be able to *sustain* giving you the help you need. People live demanding, fast-paced lives. Family members may be great at the point of diagnosis, but as time wears on, they may just get too tired. It is your responsibility to watch for this. Cut back your demands where you can. Remember to be sensitive to your family's needs and fatigue levels. *Rotate* your dependence on others as much as possible. Be aware of the symptoms of burn-out, like broken promises, lateness, and the illness of others. Emotional scenes may play out.

Third, families may give you too much of a good thing. Loving families may become smothering, controlling families. Out of concern, love, and sadness, they rise to the occasion and take charge of the situation. They take over your life and routines. They invade your privacy and personal space. In these instances, you feel great in the beginning but become unnerved, snappy, and irritable as time goes on. You want to scream, "Enough already!"

In all these cases, you must monitor your feelings about these relationships. You must look at your life and what you need now that you are ill, but be careful to respect the desires and needs of others who are serving you. The goal should be to maintain as much *independence* and *self-sufficiency* as you can. Your family may be kind, loving, giving, and attentive, but remember that they have lives, too.

Here are a few tips for successfully managing these relationships.

→ Figure out what you really need from your family.

→ Be open enough to share your physical and emotional challenges. No one can help if they don't know what to help with.

→ Ask for, but don't demand, support and help from your family.

→ Use family to escape your illness. Don't make it all work and no play. Share movies, meals, jokes, and stimulating debates.

→ Ask softly and apologetically. Receive graciously.

→ Be explicit about behaviors you like. Tell your family member if you want a pep talk or a reflective listener.

→ Ask for financial support when needed. Medical costs can be expensive; some family members would welcome the opportunity to help financially.

→ Limit contact with family members who upset you. Nobody likes everyone equally in his or her family. Get in touch with your favorite people in your family. Avoid the ones you dislike or who irritate you. Remember that you were born into your family; you didn't choose these people as your friends.

✦ Be kind to and patient with everyone who is helping, despite your feelings of irritability over the intrusion or the way people do tasks. Everyone has different ways of doing things; you must adjust to the ways of others. The quality of the end product may not meet your standards. Let rigid standards go for a while. One patient complained about how her daughter changed her bed linens and folded her towels. Now that's looking a gift horse in the mouth!

✦ Think about the other side of the coin. Your illness will have a ripple effect. What is your family's perspective? How are they feeling about all of this? What are their thoughts and fears? With the diagnosis of a serious or chronic illness, every family member will have an overwhelming fear that you are going to die. Understand that, and talk to them about it immediately. Secrets separate people. Those unspoken fears and thoughts cause isolation and alienation. Don't fall into that trap. Get those things out on the table.

✦ Remember that if you have children, you need to communicate with them about what is happening with your health. Consider the age of your child when having this discussion. Use vocabulary that is simple and age appropriate. Expect their emotional reactions. Ask them questions. Be calm, at ease, and open.

✦ Roles, responsibilities, and routines in your home will change. The use of space in your home will likely change. The normal rhythm and time of events also will probably change.

✦ Wives, remember that five types of husbands exist:

1. The **supporters** are husbands who adjust their behaviors to help you and also become your greatest cheerleaders.

2. The **cheerleaders** are husbands who give you a pep talk, but are a little short on helping or changing their routines.

3. The **sprinters** are great short-termers, but can't do the distance.

4. The **avoiders** are husbands who can't be there for you. You may hear a lot of "I have to go to work now." "I have a late business dinner." "I have a business trip." "I have a breakfast meeting."

5. The **angry** are husbands who are mad about their wife's illness and are secretly asking, "Why me?"

✦ Family members can be great patient advocates. They can help gather medical information. They can help you sort through this information and organize it. They may be opinionated, too, but, remember that treatment decisions are *your decisions*. You have the ultimate responsibility and ownership of them.

✦ Manage your relationships with family members so that you protect them from damage in the long term.

13

Friends

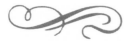

Knowledge	As written in the Book of Ecclesiasticus (6:16), "A faithful friend is the medicine of life." So said. Friends add richness, laughter, and joy to our lives. They can become a strong defense against the havoc that illness brings to your life. Friends take you out of an illness-filled world. They nurture, support, and guide you. At times, they may also let you down.
Tell Yourself	"I will successfully manage my relation-ships with friends. They can give only as much as they are capable. I must love and accept them as they are. I must be patient and accepting. Their reactions to me and my illness have most to do with themselves and little to do with me."

The nature of friendship is defined by common interests, needs, and personality styles. Now that you are ill and have physical and emotional needs that are out of the ordinary, you naturally look to friends to meet your needs. Friends play very important, and many times central, roles in the lives of patients.

✦ Friends hold the potential to help you physically. Friends commonly step up to the task by helping you to meet your daily demands. Think about how they could help you by doing things such as

- Carpooling kids
- Grocery shopping
- Helping to maintain your house
- Doing laundry
- Cooking a meal
- Running an errand
- Listening
- Advising
- Sharing an opinion.

✦ If you have a need, ask a friend if he or she can help out. Friends welcome concrete suggestions about what they can do to pitch in. Most patients find it terribly difficult to ask for help. When you make a request, begin by explaining that it is okay if the person cannot do what you request. Remember that friends realize they may be in the same boat someday.

→ Friends take you out of an illness-filled world. While your daily thoughts and worries about your health seem to weigh on you, friends provide wonderful and needed escapes. Try doing the following.

- Calling a friend on the telephone
- Having lunch or dinner with a friend
- Going to a movie
- Going on a walk
- Having a friend drive you to church
- Shopping at a mall

→ Use your time with friends to distract your thoughts away from your illness, not to draw friends into your illness.

→ Limit the amount of time you devote to discussing your diagnosis and treatments, unless the friend is helping you gather medical information or make a treatment decision. Comparisons of surgeries and treatments most often result in *more* anxiety, not less. Beware of the comparison trap.

→ Remember that no one likes to listen to complaints and self-pity. It is your responsibility to manage your conversations with friends. If you want to see a lot more of your friends, then limit your self-centered-ness and physical complaints. Many times, friends don't know what to say or do to make you feel better. If you complain too much, friends begin to feel uncomfortable and powerless when they are around

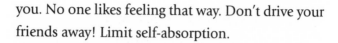

you. No one likes feeling that way. Don't drive your friends away! Limit self-absorption.

✦ Understand that your friends may be trying to make sense of your illness. Friends may conclude that you directly or indirectly are responsible for your illness. Friends may believe that you should have seen this coming, which is translated to mean that they believe they would have predicted this condition earlier if they were stricken. This protects them psychologically. Friends may degrade you in order to hold on to their belief in a just world. After all, we all learned as children that people get what they deserve. Let all these issues go. Don't get into a discussion about any of them. If comments like these are made, then reference Chapter 4.

✦ Chronic or serious illness causes anxiety in friends because it triggers a fear that it could happen to them, too.

✦ Understand that friends may believe that you are responsible for curing your illness. Ignore that belief, too.

✦ Friends should bring joy, happiness, relaxation, and relief to you. If a relationship contains conflicts or tensions, then it is up to you to either put in the energy to resolve the issues or to let go of the relationship for now.

✦ Friendships shouldn't be hard work. If contact with someone feels like that, something is probably wrong.

✦ Avoid intrusive people.

✦ Avoid those people who give you pitying attitudes. Copers don't have time for pity.

✦ You should know that some friendships end or fall apart when a chronic or serious illness hits. In most cases, when a friend drops out of your life after you've become ill, it is not because of you. You've probably seen people who just cannot visit a hospital or funeral home. They can't handle seeing your pain. They over-identify with you. You will feel disappointed, angry, and sad. If you want to resolve the situation, consider the following suggestions.

  – Take steps to contact the friend. Write a note or make a phone call. Ignore the fact that they've disappeared from your life. Sometimes, it's just a matter of breaking the ice.

  – Sometimes you may not be able to get over your hurt feelings. This is truly your loss. It's up to you to try to respond to your friend, despite your illness. Put yourself in your friend's position, based on what you know about him or her. Perhaps a rational explanation exists for the behavior.

- You may openly ask your friend about his or her absence. Be careful not to come across as argumentative or cutting. Like most of life, you reap the rewards of hard work. The key is to choose whether you want to invest more in a relationship or live with the status quo.

→ Friends aren't always perfect. They aren't predictable. They may not know what to say or do when you are ill. Help them out. Open a dialogue with them.

→ Remember that when you share intimacy, you risk feeling disappointed with how others respond. However, you may get boundless rewards. Friendships may blossom in new and unexpected ways.

→ Don't be fooled that others who are also ill are in a position to befriend, support, and nurture you. *Friendships born from common misery are probably only fleeting company.*

→ Practice restraint and remember that time may change your opinion and perspective. Don't judge your friends too hastily.

→ Misfortune has a way of showing you who your true friends are and what they are made of.

14

Giving Thanks

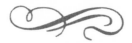

Knowledge	You should always give thanks to others for their efforts, support, generosity, and acts of kindness. No act by others should be ignored or taken for granted. The most important thing you can do to maintain your supportive relationships is to give thanks.
Tell Yourself	"I will always acknowledge and thank others for their physical and emotional support. I will not take others for granted. I will make extra effort to thank my closest and most dependable supporters."

↬ Consider using the following words.

 – "Your kindness warms my heart."

 – "Your words really cheer me up."

- "Thanks for taking time from your busy schedule to help out."
- "Your help is so appreciated. I never could have done it without you."
- "You'll never know how much I appreciate your help. Thanks."
- "You're a gem!"
- "When I think of your generosity, I am over-whelmed."
- "You fill my day with joy. Thanks."
- "Thanks for helping me, despite your busy life."
- "Thanks for creating a ripple in my life. You take me out of boredom."
- "Thanks for the merriment and good cheer!"
- "I really enjoy your company. It takes me away from illness."

✦ Consider doing the following.

- Baking cookies and writing a thank-you note.
- Sending flowers.
- Creating a craft, if you're talented in that way.
- Sending a book.
- Telephoning to say thanks.
- Sending a card.
- Giving the giver a hug.

15

Creating Hope

Knowledge	Hope is a dream. Hope is created in your thoughts. You define a future goal, direct your actions to achieve that goal, and have an expectation that you will reach that goal.
Tell Yourself	"I will create my dream. I will define a goal and take steps to reach my goal. I will hope for those things that I expect to achieve. Hope will bring me joy, happiness, and self-fulfillment."

What is hope? How might you create hopefulness in your life? Only you may define things to hope for. Some healers believe that hope leads to better coping and better health. Others claim that if your health improves or you adapt to your illness, you will experience more hope.

Hope involves focusing on the attainment of something you want in your future. You should hope for things that you generally believe you can attain. The more hope you can create in your life, the happier and more productive you will be on a daily basis. You have the ability to create hope in your attitudes and thoughts throughout your day.

→ Hope is awakening a dream that you create.

→ Hope may be a belief that you can and will transcend your illness.

→ Hope is realized when you achieve a goal. Set your goals, but make them realistic.

→ Hope will sustain you through physical pain and grief.

→ Hope will conquer your cowardice.

→ Hope will fuel you for your struggle against lethargy and self-pity.

→ Hope is experienced when you exert effort. Hope does not just happen. It is created.

→ Defy the negative impact of this illness on your life. You must defy your illness each day.

→ Be flexible regarding the expectations you have of yourself. If you are defiant without being flexible, you may end up defeated, exhausted, and feeling like a failure. Give yourself permission to let go of certain things, but be sure you are pushing yourself to produce to your maximum extent.

✦ Compartmentalize. You don't have to be a sickly patient 24 hours a day.

✦ Pace yourself. Manage your activities so that you'll have energy to expend when and where you want. All your activities should be conscious choices.

✦ Manage your time and resources to meet your goals.

✦ Find activities that will take your mind off your physical challenges. Don't choose activities that create more problems for you.

✦ Focus on gaining control of your routines and daily responsibilities.

✦ Again, don't think about or focus on your disease prognosis. If your thoughts drift to your prognostic statistic, assure yourself that you will side with the winners.

✦ Giving to others somehow makes us all feel vital and alive. Consider volunteering to do something for others, even if you have a chronic or life-threatening illness.

✦ Being needed gives us definition and purpose. Define yourself! Become needed.

- Maintain a focus on your purpose and mission in life. We all have purpose. Staying in tune with your life mission will fuel your hopefulness.
- Focus on short-term pleasures—a birthday, an anniversary, a holiday, or a graduation.
- Find things that you believe will help your health—like a good diet, vitamins, or exercise. Commit yourself to a healing way of life.
- Remember that no one can predict with absolute certainty how quickly your disease may progress or how long you are going to live. Constantly tell yourself that you will be a treatment success.
- Transcend the effects of illness and treatments. Enjoy each moment of life.

Bibliography

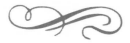

American Cancer Society: www.cancer.org

Aspinwall, L.G., & MacNamara, A. (2005). Taking positive changes seriously. *Cancer, 104*(11), 2549–2556.

Cancer Survivors Network: www.acscsn.org

Doyle, N., & Kelly, D. (2005). "So what happens now?" Issues in cancer survival and rehabilitation. *Clinical Effectiveness in Nursing, 9*(3–4), 147–153.

Gullatte, M.M. (Ed.). (2007). *Clinical guide to antineoplastic therapy: A chemotherapy handbook* (2nd ed.). Pittsburgh, PA: Oncology Nursing Society.

Hansen, F., & Sawatzky, J.V. (2008). Stress in patients with lung cancer: A human response to illness. *Oncology Nursing Forum, 35*(2), 217–223.

Haylock, P.J. (2006). The shifting paradigm of cancer care. *American Journal of Nursing, 106*(3), 16–19.

Jansen, J., van Weert, J., van Dulmen, S., Heeren, T., & Bensing, J. (2007). Patient education about treatment in cancer care: An overview of the literature on older patients' needs. *Cancer Nursing, 30*(4), 251–260.

Kattlove, H., & Winn, R.J. (2003). Ongoing care of patients after primary treatment for their cancer. *CA: A Cancer Journal for Clinicians, 53*(3), 172–196.

Lamond, D., & Thompson, C. (2000). Intuition and analysis in decision making and choice. *Journal of Nursing Scholarship, 32*(3), 411–414.

Ligibel, J.A. (2007). Can lifestyle choices influence breast cancer risk and prognosis? *Journal of Supportive Oncology, 5*(2), 60.

MacBride, S.K., & Whyte, F. (1998). Survivorship and the cancer follow-up clinic. *European Journal of Cancer Care, 7*(1), 47–55.

National Cancer Institute: www.cancer.gov

Penson, R.T., Gu, F., Harris, S., Thiel, M.M., Lawton, N., Fuller, A.F., et al. (2007). Hope. *Oncologist, 12*(9), 1105–1113.

Schover, L.R. (1991). The impact of breast cancer on sexuality, body image, and intimate relationships. *CA: A Cancer Journal for Clinicians, 41*(2), 112–120.

Sepucha, K., & Belkora, J. (2007). Putting shared decision making to work in breast and prostate cancers: Tools for community oncologists. *Community Oncology, 4*(11), 685–689, 691.

Simmons, L.A. (2007). Self-perceived burden in cancer patients. *Cancer Nursing, 30*(5), 405–411.

Vachon, M. (2006). Psychosocial distress and coping after cancer treatment: How clinicians can assess distress and which interventions are appropriate—what we know and what we don't. *Cancer Nursing, 29*(2), 26–31.

van Weert, E., Hoekstra-Weebers, J., Otter, R., Postema, K., Sanderman, R., & van der Schans, C. (2006). Cancer-related fatigue: Predictors and effects of rehabilitation. *Oncologist, 11*(2), 184–196.

Online Resources

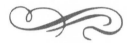

American Cancer Society. (n.d.). *Coping with treatment.* Retrieved April 3, 2008, from http://www.cancer.org/docroot/HOME/pff/PFF_2.asp

Cancer.Net Editorial Board. (2005, July 11). *Supporting a friend who has cancer.* Retrieved April 3, 2008, from http://www.cancer.net/patient/Library/Cancer.Net+Features/Guidance+and+Support/Supporting+a+Friend+Who+Has+Cancer#mainContentidmain Content

Cancer Family Care. (n.d.). *You can help when your friend has cancer.* Retrieved April 3, 2008, from http://www.cancerfamilycare.org/content/view/28/62/

Cleveland Clinic Foundation. (2006, December 5). *Cancer and exercise.* Retrieved April 3, 2008, from http://www.revolutionhealth.com/conditions/breast-cancer/exercise-overview

Coping With Cancer magazine. [Subscription information available at http://www.copingmag.com/cancer/index.html]

Creagan, E.T. (2007, July 16). *Cancer diagnosis? Advice for dealing with what comes next.* Message posted to http://www.mayoclinic.com/health/cancer-diagnosis/HQ00379

Dr. Kataria School of Laughter Yoga. (n.d.). *Power of positive affirmations.* Retrieved April 3, 2008, from http://www.laughteryoga.org/positive-affirmations.php

Fury, M.G. (2006, October). *Diagnosis.* Retrieved April 3, 2008, from http://www.merck.com/mmhe/sec15/ch181/ch181c.html

Johns Hopkins Avon Foundation Breast Center. (n.d.). *I'm done with my treatment—now what?* Retrieved April 3, 2008, from http://www.hopkinsbreastcenter.org/library/diagnosis_treatment/post_treatment.shtml

Mayo Foundation for Medical Education and Research. (2007, September 10). *Cancer diagnosis: 10 tips for coping.* Retrieved April 3, 2008, from http://www.mayoclinic.com/health/cancer-diagnosis/HQ01306

Mayo Foundation for Medical Education and Research. (2007, October 2). *Cancer survivors: Reconnecting with family and friends after treatment.* Retrieved April 3, 2008, from http://www.mayoclinic.com/health/cancer-survivor/CA00072

National Cancer Institute. (2008, March 6). *Coping with cancer.* Retrieved April 3, 2008, from http://www.nci.nih.gov/cancertopics/coping

National Cancer Institute. (n.d.). *Taking time: Support for people with cancer.* Retrieved April 3, 2008, from http://cancernet.nci.nih.gov/cancertopics/takingtime